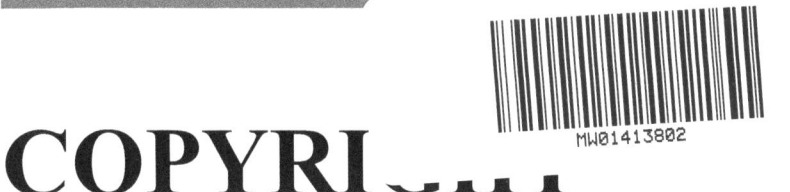

COPYRIGHT

Copyright © 2018 by Dalal Davilla

All rights reserved. No part of this publication may be reproduced, distributed, or transmitted in any form or by any means, including photocopying, recording, or other electronic or mechanical methods, without the prior written permission of the publisher, except in the case of brief quotations embodied in critical reviews and certain other noncommercial uses permitted by copyright law. For permission requests, write to the publisher, addressed "Attention: Permissions Coordinator," at the email address books@dalaldavilla.com.

For other information, please visit :

www.dalaldavilla.com

TABLE OF CONTENTS

Copyright 1

Table of Contents 2

about 5

Chapter 1 7

    Learning About Yoga 7

        1.1 Introduction to Yoga 8

        1.2 Benefits of Yoga Practice 9

        1.3 Yoga Styles 11

        1.4 Alternative Fundamentals of Yoga to Adapt them to Daily Routines 12

Chapter 2 14

    Integration 14

        2.1 Knowing your Body 15

Table of Contents

 2.2 Acceptance and Fluidity in Movements 17

Chapter 3 18

 Yoga for Beginners 18

  3.1 Steps to Start a Yoga Practice 19

  3.2 Tools to Strengthen the Mind, Body and Spirit 19

  3.3 Materials that Facilitate Yoga Practice 20

Chapter 4 21

 Pranayama 21

  4.1 Breathing Exercises 22

  4.2 Meditation and Introspection 26

Chapter 5 28

 Yoga Poses: Asanas 28

  5.1 Yoga Poses for Beginners 30

  5.2 Yoga Poses to Warm and Tone the Body 38

  5.3 Yoga Poses for Balance 45

  5.4 Yoga poses for Relaxation and Stimulation of Emotions 54

Chapter 6 63

 Healthy Food for Yoguis 63

  6.1 Importance of a Balanced Diet 64

Table of Contents

    6.2 The Gunas 64

Chapter 7 70

    Physical Transformation 70

    7.1 Yoga Integral Alternative for Weight Loss 71

    7.2 Increased Self-Esteem: Trust and Security 75

Chapter 8 76

    The Moment is Here and Now 76

Chapter 9 79

    Positive Aspects of Performing Physical Activities 79

    9.1 Positive Effects Provided by the Constant Practice of Yoga and Exercise 80

    9.2 Welfare and for the environment 83

Chapter 10 86

    Mindfulness 86

ABOUT

This material has been created with the focus of providing detailed information on the philosophy of yoga and the practice that is carried out with the aim of benefiting the lives of millions of people, in order to motivate millions of hearts and inspire their will to start practicing this discipline millenary that provides physical, mental and spiritual health.

Yoga is designed for everyone: children, teenagers, women with curves, men, and elderly, there are no limits of age, time or borders, it is time to conquer the best version of us.

Yoga is a complementary tool which provides physical, mental and spiritual well-being. The present e-book is especially designed for all girls with curves in the world who decide to undertake the integral practice of Yoga that leads us to acceptance of ourselves with those we have, desire and what we are.

When I was a teenager I felt many complexes because when running my whole body jumped vigorously making me clumsy with the movements or in swimming I did not feel comfortable wearing a bathing suit, with the hikes I felt that there was not a seat big enough to hold my butt in reality always I had an excuse not to create exercise habits, my body stood out for the volume, I am a curvy girl, beautiful and intelligent but with insecurities

about

for my body, for being different, with the passage of time I knew the practice of yoga, experiencing that feeling of equality, it did not matter to be different, there were no requirements to make a class just need a mat and pay attention to the breathing and movements of my body, sounds easy and really is.

The practice of yoga awakened my conscience, every time I progressed in practice it was an advance in life, I gained security, confidence, self-esteem, with each meditation I felt as I fell more and more in love with myself, with my curves, with my strength . Yoga leads us to paths of introspection developing the union of all that we are body, mind and spirit, creating the discernment of what we think, say and do in order to connect with that superior power that is hidden in each of us and we connects with the divinity.

I invite you to enjoy these informative lines, made with a lot of love thought about you beautiful girl with curves, it is possible to motivate ourselves to do great things.

"Namaste"

CHAPTER 1

Learning About Yoga

Chapter 1

1.1 Introduction to Yoga

Yoga is an integral discipline of the body, mind and spirit that consists of directing attention to our thoughts, words, movements and acts through sequences of physical and respiratory exercises that provide well-being, strength and psychophysical conditioning. Yoga is also considered as one of the most outstanding methods to look inwards. Yoga is born from the Sanskrit language in the Hindu culture which means "union" or integration of the individual conscience with the universal conscience (soul or spirit) its content is universal and act for all.

Note: Yoga practice is often confused with religion but it is not necessary to believe in a specific religion or god to learn the yoga teachings.

The practice of yoga consists of performing postures with therapeutic purposes known as asanas, that help rehabilitate the body's posture and maintain optimal functioning of the internal organs and metabolism, in addition to strengthening the body, toning and contributing to weight loss, flexibility and health. Followed by the practice of Pranayamas (breathing techniques) also known as "control of prana" (vital energy), meditation that encourage the development of awareness and control of breathing, emotions and moods. Yoga encourages the fulfillment of moral values that contribute to well-being with all living beings, which is why it is considered as a holistic and integral practice.

"To release the potential of your mind, body and soul, you must first expand your imagination. Things are always created twice: first in the workshop of the mind and then in reality".

-Robin Sharma.

1.2 Benefits of Yoga Practice

Part of the Benefits of Yoga is to contribute to the mental health of each individual:

- ✓ Improve concentration and focus
- ✓ Create positive habits
- ✓ Contribute to the detachment of toxic emotions (depression, anxiety)
- ✓ Increase self-esteem
- ✓ Develop security, confidence, determination and will
- ✓ Overcoming the barriers of fear
- ✓ Awakening of consciousness

Yoga is an excellent stimulant of emotions, this contributes favorably to the acceptance of the body, mastery of thoughts and sensations, with the help of meditation and breathing techniques.

Chapter 1

Benefits of Physical Yoga:

Doing yoga postures (asanas) contributes to:

- ✓ Make your body and mind more flexible
- ✓ Condition the body
- ✓ Develop pulmonary and cardiovascular resistance
- ✓ Align body posture
- ✓ Contribute to weight loss
- ✓ Toning the body and regulating the appetite

Spiritual Benefits:

- ✓ Stimulate faith and hope
- ✓ Foster compassionate love
- ✓ Develop the belief in oneself
- ✓ Connect the human essence with the universe

Social benefits:

- ✓ Socialize harmoniously
- ✓ Stimulate emotions
- ✓ Encouraging communication and acceptance of cultural diversity

Chapter 1

"You have to do yoga for the pleasure of doing it and enjoy its benefits."

-B.K.S Iyengar.

1.3 Yoga Styles

This discipline includes several classic and historical styles of practice that guide each individual to develop their greatest potentialities and find what is often hidden within their being. Yoga is for everyone and this book is especially for all girls with curves that deepen the practice with devotion and enthusiasm.

Then the classic yoga trails:

- <u>Raja Yoga:</u> Is the most known today, which is related to the control of the mind and body through meditation, breathing and physical work.
- <u>Hatha Yoga:</u> That is to say the yoga of the postures, called asanas whose fundamental objective is to purify the body.
- <u>Karma Yoga:</u> Is the yoga of service performed selflessly, without attachment to the results.
- <u>Bhakti Yoga:</u> Is the path of love and includes rituals, ceremonies and songs, it is attractive for devotional and mystical people.
- <u>Mantra Yoga:</u> Is to center the consciousness in our interior by means of the repetition of universal sounds, for example the OM.

- ✓ <u>The Guiana Yoga:</u> Which is the intellectual study of texts, whoever practices it must have mastered the other techniques and must have great understanding and will before knowledge and wisdom.

These categories of yoga are the roots of the practice that today is taught worldwide. Experts or instructors integrate methods, experiences and studies of the great masters of the history of yoga to provide their students the right knowledge to transcend time, age and often obstacles that the mind sows in consciousness. Some of the most practiced types of yoga are: *Jivamukti Yoga, Ashtanga Yoga, Dharma Yoga, Vinyasa Yoga and Kundalini Yoga.*

"Healthy people and plants produce abundant flowers and fruits. Similarly, a healthy person smiles and is happy like the rays of the sun".

-B.K. S Iyengar.

1.4 Alternative Fundamentals of Yoga to Adapt them to Daily Routines

The philosophy of yoga is based on the study of the Yoga Sutra which are the set of aphorisms that are taught in the practice of yoga by encouraging attention to our actions to create union and discernment with ourselves and in coexistence with the world.

Chapter 1

Ashtanga yoga or 8-step yoga encompasses a set of complementary techniques that constitute the entire practice of yoga.

- ✓ The yamas (moral restrictions, such as non-violence, truth of speech, act and thought, not stealing, moderation and non-possessiveness)
- ✓ The niyamas (purity, contentment, austerity, the study of sacred texts, and the permanent awareness of divinity)
- ✓ The asanas (postures)
- ✓ Pranayama (adequate breathing)
- ✓ Pratyahara (the recollection of the senses)
- ✓ Dharana (concentration for meditation)
- ✓ Dyana (meditation and contemplation)
- ✓ Samadi (supra-consciousness).

The more you become involved in the practice of yoga, the greater the physical, mental and spiritual progress that can be experienced. Taking time to breathe slowly, respecting the individuality of others and moving the whole body with prudence will be part of the positive habits to be experienced with the practice of yoga, which will make easier to relate to others on a day to day basis.

CHAPTER 2

Integration

Chapter 2

2.1 Knowing your Body

The human body is totally diverse in height, diameter, contours, curves, weight and volume. Many times the excuses for not exercising come from physical conditions such as: I am fat, very tall, very low, weak, skinny and so on. In the practice of yoga there are no physical or mental limitations, all type of bodies are fit to perform a sequence of asanas, the important thing is to respect the body that each one possesses, since many by wanting to make the postures as the instructors or teachers are forcing and attacking the body causing injuries and even disappointments, constant practice is what develops strength, flexibility and balance.

<u>Note:</u> It is important to have a sense of belonging with ourselves, if you are a girl with curves please do not be afraid or pity to use your movements with ease and confidence, yoga stimulates inner beauty and multiplies smiles.

Do you have any symptoms or medical condition?

The practice of yoga contributes to the rehabilitation of the body, physical and mental health, however there are contraindications when performing inverted or contorted postures for people with asthmatic states, blood pressure, glaucoma, chronic migraines, arthritis, among others. It is important to know the functioning of the body and practice with a

Chapter 2

professional in yoga that can offer options when performing the practice and ensure the enjoyment of the therapeutic benefits of yoga.

What are your weaknesses?

Knowledge is the door of power. Knowing the physical realities you have is the first step to achieve the positive transformation of the body, mind and spirit, since at the time of recognizing the physical and mental weaknesses, it will be more effective to transform them into virtues.

What are your strengths?

The physical and mental strengths allow to reach the development of the maximum potential that one can have. This consists in highlighting the virtues that are available as: disposition, encouragement, confidence, resistance and other positive aspects.

"Who finds his happiness in the inner vision of Knowledge, has his senses and joyful heart subject, due to the experience of his own inner life. Only then can he be recognized as a Yogi in harmony. Once reached this state, for him, gold has no more value than the stones of the earth".

-Krishna. Bhagavad Gita.

2.2 Acceptance and Fluidity in Movements

Once the body and mental awareness is created, focusing attention to achieve well-being will be much more fun, since with focus, determination and desire, work will be done on physical conditioning, strengthening of thoughts and flexibility of character. Yoga provides multiple benefits in the life and environment of its practitioners.

The acceptance of who we are and the tools we have to develop the practice is fundamental to advance in the flow of movement and body expression. Many times beautiful girls with curves or of small size usually have complexes because their bodies are different, discouraging them, however in yoga the curves and the size have no relevance, the power comes with the attitude and the desire to reach the maximum potential of their bodies and the control of thoughts.

CHAPTER 3

Yoga for Beginners

3.1 Steps to Start a Yoga Practice

The first step to begin to experience the wonderful benefits of yoga is to have the desire for transformation and reach states of calm and control.

The second big step is to find the guide of a good instructor or teacher who can meet your needs.

The following steps will depend on the practice, interest and perseverance of each person.

I am sure that the next ones will be transformers and revolutionaries in your life.

3.2 Tools to Strengthen the Mind, Body and Spirit

- Attitude
- Will
- Mental and spiritual strength
- Time
- You want

The main tool of power comes from the mind, which is why yoga places so much emphasis on the integration of thoughts and attitudes.

3.3 Materials that Facilitate Yoga Practice

In Yoga are different types of practice, which can stimulate the efficiency and harmony of each individual according to their needs and requirements. At the time of performing sequences of Yoga as the props that are used to perform yoga with greater comfort and ease, granting alignment and support in the movements and thus bring the practitioners closer with each asana little by little.

Examples:

- Yoga Mat
- Box (cushions)
- Belts
- Blocks
- Chairs.

CHAPTER 4

Pranayama

Chapter 4

4.1 Breathing Exercises

Breathing is a vital and natural process in living beings, consists of the entrance of oxygen to the body and the release of carbon dioxide from it. In the practice of Yoga, learning to control breathing is as important as maintaining a correct posture, this provides greater physical skills and mastery of emotions.

Types of Pranayamas - Breathing Techniques:

Abdominal breathing.

Normally in the first yoga classes attention is directed to how we breathe in order to ensure the practice correctly and awaken the physical consciousness of each individual, developing the control of body and mind.

Preparation 1:

Savasana: On a yoga mat, lie on your back, with your body fully supported on the floor, your feet are separated by the width of the hips, the spine in a straight line with head, hands at the sides of the body with palms towards Above, the muscles and thoughts relax while you seek to inhale and exhale deeply and slowly.

To recognize how the incoming air is distributed with the inhalations, support hands on the abdomen, overdraw fingers to cover the

Chapter 4

area between the lower ribs and the pelvic area. Inhale rhythmically through the nose for three or four times and exhale during the same period. Every time you inhale, observe that the abdomen rises, and every time you exhale appreciate how the navel goes inward. When breathing is understood, increase the permanence of exhalation.

Place weight on the abdomen (a book, a folded towel or a small cushion) resting the arms on the floor. Continue to breathe rhythmically, the abdomen ascends when inhaling and descends when exhaling.

Keep the weight on the abdomen, cross the arms with force on the chest and try to touch the shoulder blades. This pressure on the rib cage will give greater abdominal strength, trying to keep the chest from moving during inhalation, allowing the abdomen to expand more and more with breathing.

"Forget the past, because it is outside your domain. Forget the future, because it is beyond your reach. Control the present. Live supremely well now. That is the way of wisdom".

-Paramahansa Yogananda.

Complete breathing (abdominal, thoracic and clavicular).

Chapter 4

Preparation 2:

Sukhasana: Sitting cross-legged, in meditation posture or simple pose.

In complete yogic breathing, inhalation occurs in three stages:

- First the diaphragm moves down into the abdomen, bringing air to the lower part of the lungs
- Then the intercostal muscles expand the rib cage and push the air to the middle part of the lungs
- Finally, the air reaches the upper part of the chest. This is called clavicle breathing.

Sitting cross-legged, resting one hand on the abdomen and the other on the ribs. In order to recognize the abdominal movements that occur with inspiration. Perform a complete abdominal inhalation, continue with the inhalation raising the rib cage, keep inhaling to fill the upper end of the lungs, enhancing the clavicles. Make sure to maintain abdominal expansion at all times and not to raise the shoulders towards the ears. Then begin to exhale from the abdomen slowly, expel air from the chest and finally relax the area surrounding the clavicles.

By mastering the complete yogic breathing, seek to adapt the breathing in Tadasa or mountain posture (standing fully erect body), and so

Chapter 4

little by little go creating the integration of the conscious breath in each posture and activities that you perform in the day to day.

Breathing Ujjayi:

In a comfortable position (standing, lying on your back or sitting), release the air you have in your body, with a deep exhalation, while paying full attention to the manifestations of the mind (thoughts) and bodily sensations.

When inhaling through the nostrils the air first fills the stomach, then the rib cage and then the upper part of the chest. The air that has been inhaled passes through the throat generating a slight contraction of the glottis that is to say of the muscles of the posterior part of the base of the neck, next to the root of the clavicle. When exhaling through the nose, a uniform sound is produced, similar to the waves of the sea.

The sound that is experienced is the result of the contraction of the vocal cords which causes the air to vibrate (when inhaled) in front of the glottis and behind it (when exhaling).

Repeat this breathing exercise as many times as necessary to create awareness of the breathing rhythm.

The Ujjayi breathing develops the lung capacity of the human being. It stimulates the nervous system completely, generating calm and serenity,

Chapter 4

in the same way it helps to dissolve the mental fluctuations, favoring the concentration, the state of permanence, the good internal functioning of the body, among others.

Recommendations

- Keep eyes closed
- Relax facial muscles
- If you choose to perform this exercise sitting comfortably, maintain the straightness of the spine.

4.2 Meditation and Introspection

Meditation is a personal experience that induces the individual to inquire into their interior, recognizing the noise of the mind, thoughts and sensations. Yoga favors holistically in all aspects of life, guiding people to perform meditation techniques before, during and after the practice of asanas, which contributes to the well-being of the conscience and the body, generating harmony and tranquility in the thoughts and acts. With constant practice and discipline yoga develops positive states of consciousness, acceptance and respect for life and neighbor making possible a healthier and pleasant internal and external coexistence.

Guided Meditation:

Chapter 4

Sitting in a comfortable position close your eyes and perform continuous breathing exercises, channeling thoughts and sensations. Relax facial muscles and the body. Pay full attention to the thoughts that come and go. Keep your breath conscious while identifying the priorities of your mind, good thoughts, bad thoughts, questions, doubts, focus your attention on positive and overcoming phrases in order to get good energy and concentrate on releasing the restlessness of the mind. Feel and pay attention on the slow and slow breathing that gradually calm your conscience until you manage to silence your mind and simply feel how the air enters through your nasal fossals nourishing each cell and exhale as you exhale each worry.

Perform this exercise daily for as long as it is necessary for you.

Note: The biggest challenge of meditation will be to maintain a serene position in the face of explosive or uncomfortable circumstances.

"Now, after having done the previous preparation through life itself and other practices, begins the study and practice of Yoga".

-Patanjali. Yoga Sutras.

CHAPTER 5

Yoga Poses: Asanas

Chapter 5

Asanas are postures that are made throughout the practice of yoga in coordination of slow and conscious breathing.

With these 20 basic asanas that will be explained below, you can start a harmonious yoga practice ideal for all those who wish to enjoy the multiple benefits of the poses. It is a simple and fun continuous sequence that can be performed in 25 minutes, designed especially for girls and boys with curves, who desire to experience the transformation of their body, strengthen the mind and harmonize the spirit.

The fluid movements that develop with the asanas are part of your body expression, please respect the conditions of your body, it is normal to maintain greater balance on one side than the other, that the left hip is more flexible than the right or vice versa, Each body has its strengths and weaknesses, balance and dexterity are acquired with constant practice, as well as developing relaxation at all times, weight loss, emotional control and others, little by little of anger enjoying the infinite benefits of yoga, depends on you and your perseverance. It is important to emphasize that in order to give the body the therapeutic benefits of each posture, the time of permanence must be at least 3 breaths.

Note: Always perform both sides of the body, even if the instructions are explained on one side only.

Chapter 5

"Yoga does not take us away from reality or the responsibilities of daily life, but puts our feet firmly and resolutely in the practical field of experience. We do not transcend our lives; we return to the lives we have left behind in the hope of something better".

-Donna Farhi.

5.1 Yoga Poses for Beginners

Mountain Pose – Tadasana

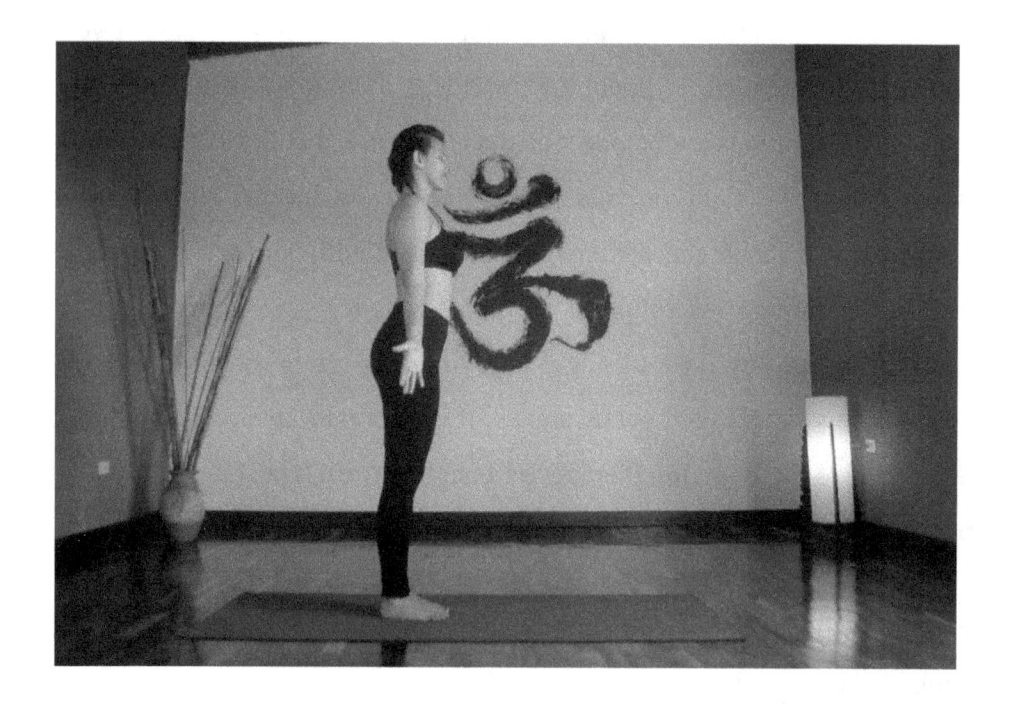

Chapter 5

Standing the body weight is distributed between both soles of the feet. Arms go to the side of the body, relaxing shoulders, with the spine as straight as you can. Notice the straight line that goes from the crown of my head to the sacrum. The abdomen remains active and contracted, the conscious breathing is present inhaled, exhaling gently directing the attention towards the inside, perceiving the energy level emanating from the body.

Benefits

- Ensures a perfect alignment of the spine
- Improves body posture
- Mitigates back pain
- Contribute to the flow of blood throughout the body.

Recommendations

- Relax shoulders and release tensions
- Concentrate on breathing.

High Lunge Pose - Utthita Ashwa Sanchalanasana

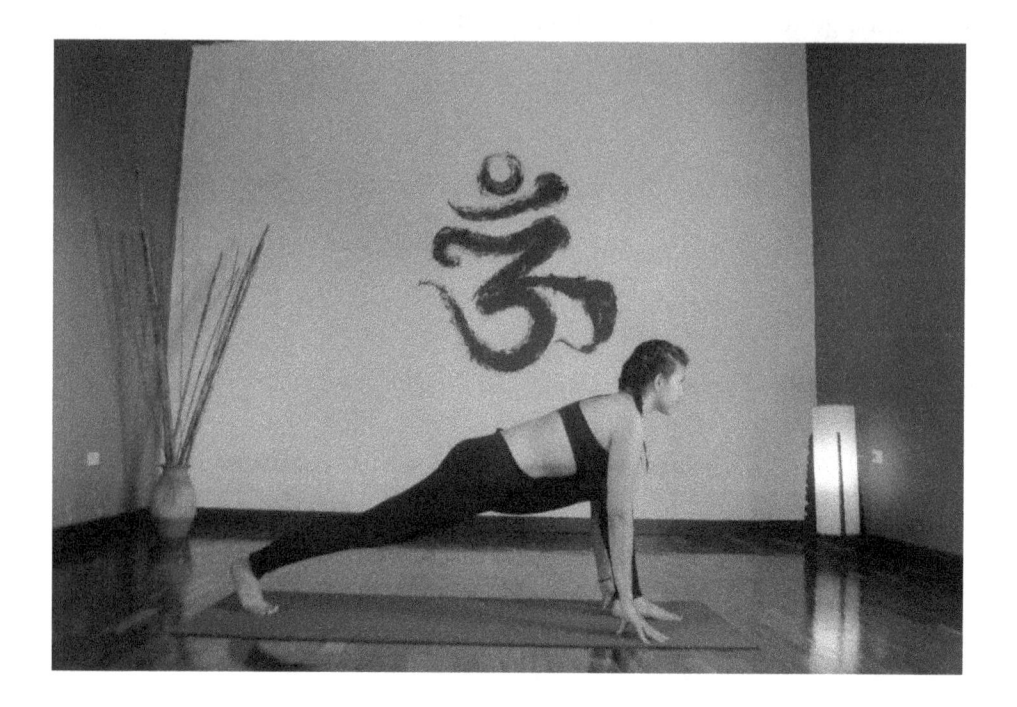

Also known as the runner posture. The left foot goes backwards with the leg well extended, while the right foot is ahead with the knee flexes both hands are supported on the mat. The gaze rests on the horizon, the column is as straight as possible. Perform the posture with both sides of the body.

Benefits

- Strengthens the calves and thighs
- Toning arms and abdomen
- Contributes to the opening of the hips.

Chapter 5

Recommendations

- Do not support body weight on the bent knee
- If your hands do not touch the ground, help yourself with some yoga blocks.

Downward Facing Dog - Adho Mukha Svanasana

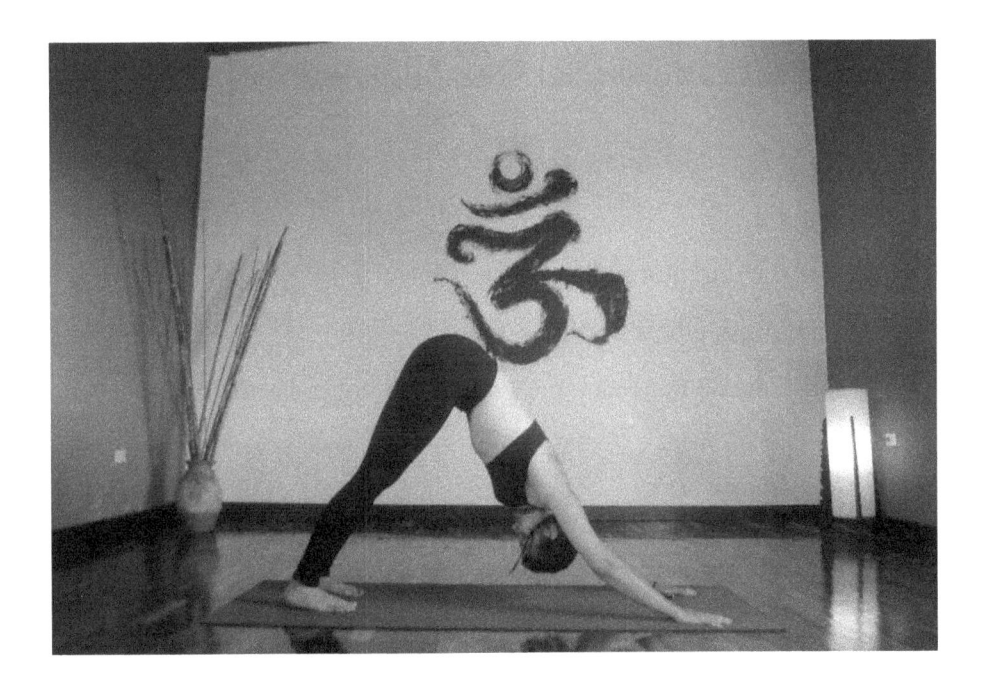

On the yoga mat support the knees flexing and hands with extended arms take the look towards the navel and raise little high on the coccyx, the knees are separated from the floor spreading the legs, the heels seek to lean on the ground making a V inverted with the body.

Note: It is important to note that each body is different therefore if you feel pain when extending your knees, please do not look to extend them, maintain a subtle flexion and concentration on breathing. Keep 5 breaths.

Benefits

- Contributes to the relaxation of the body
- Stimulates the blood flow of the blood and oxygenate the brain
- Strengthens adductors, articulation of the knees and ankles.

Recommendations

- Avoid the curvature of the back
- Do not press elbows or knees
- If the heels do not reach the ground, do not press the body.

Chair Pose – Utkatasana

Chapter 5

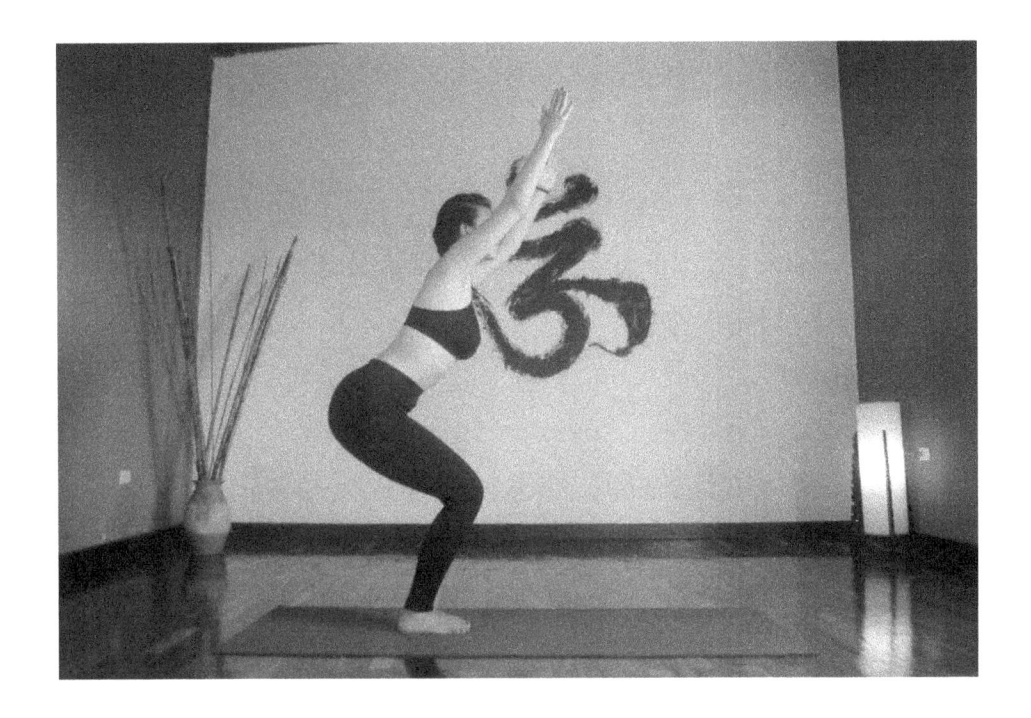

Standing perform a deep bending of knees while the weight of the body is distributed on both feet, pay attention not to exceed the toes. The arms and the back of the body inclined diagonally at 45 ° from the ground, the abdomen contracts and the buttocks go back, the focus is on the space created between both hands. It is really imagining sitting in a chair, but this time the spine stays in a straight position and every part of the body is active.

Benefits

- Deep stretch of shoulders and arms
- Strengthens the abdominal muscles
- Add resistance to the thighs, knees and ankles

- Stimulates the digestive organs

Recommendations

- If you have any pain or discomfort in your knees, refrain from doing this position
- If you suffer from cervical not force the gaze up, but rather semi-flex elbows and keep a fixed point on the ground
- Be cautious if your body shows any headache or vertigo
- Abstain people with blood pressure.

Triangle Pose - Trikonasana

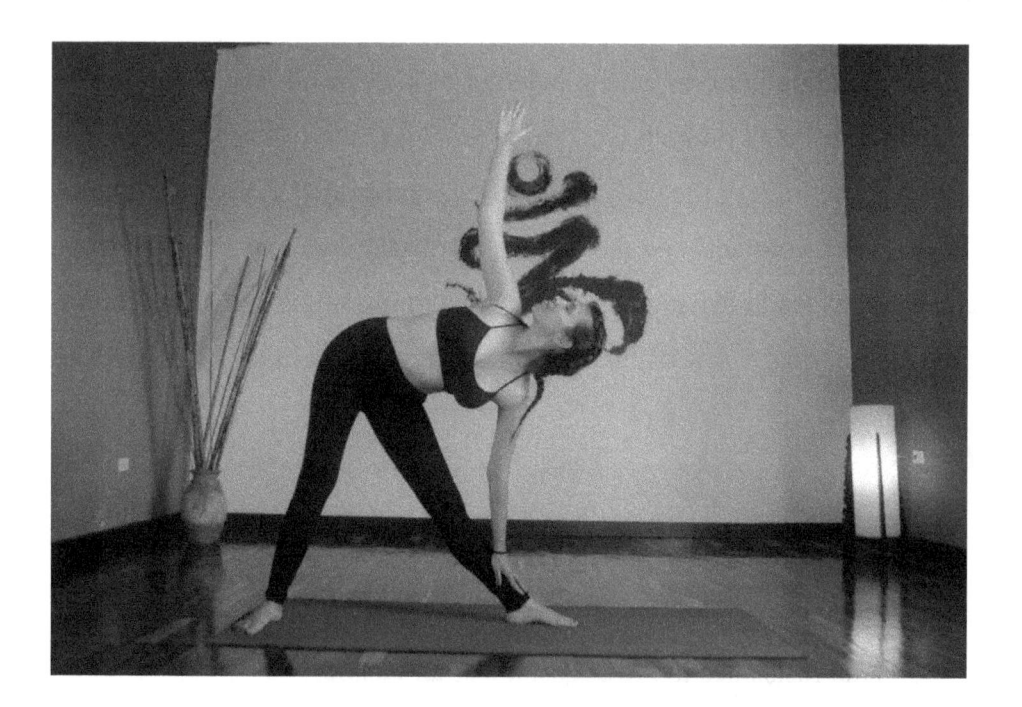

Chapter 5

Stand with your legs spread shoulder width apart. Take a deep inhale while raising both arms to the sides so that they are parallel with the floor, exhale and with one foot perpendicular to the other, a lateral flexion of the hip is made.

Support the left hand on the ankle, calf or thigh, while the free arm goes up vertically with the palm of the hand facing forward, to look at the ring finger that is on top.

To the extent that the posture is assumed, control the breathing in order to deepen the same.

Perform complementary side.

Benefits

- Relieves back pain
- Stretches and strengthens thighs, knees and ankles
- Contributes to the opening of the chest
- Stimulates concentration.

Recommendations

- If you feel discomfort in the neck, look towards the floor
- Contract abdomen to ensure alignment of the pose
- Do not exaggerate the opening of the legs.

Chapter 5

5.2 Yoga Poses to Warm and Tone the Body

Goddess Pose - Utkata Konasana

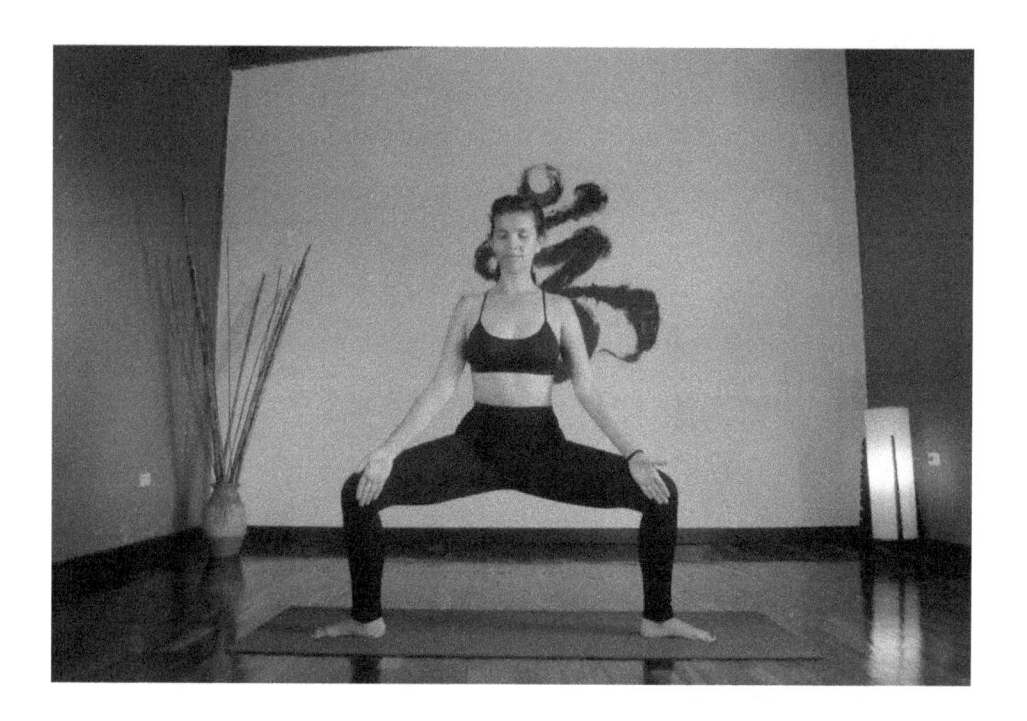

Keeping the legs open in the anterior position, the toes are turned slightly outward, as indicated by the corners of the mat, with the help of the inhalation the knees are flexed, the buttocks and abdomen are kept contracted and firm. The back stays in a straight line and the face relaxed. Let your hands rest on your knees or you can bring them together to the center of your chest.

Benefits

Chapter 5

- Stimulates the balance of the body
- Toning column, abdomen and legs
- Contributes to the resistance of the body and the mind
- Makes the pelvic floor more flexible.

Recommendations

- Pay attention that the knees do not pass the toes
- Do not pull out the tail, rotate the hip forward
- Keep the spine straight.

Variation Warrior I - Virabhadrasana I

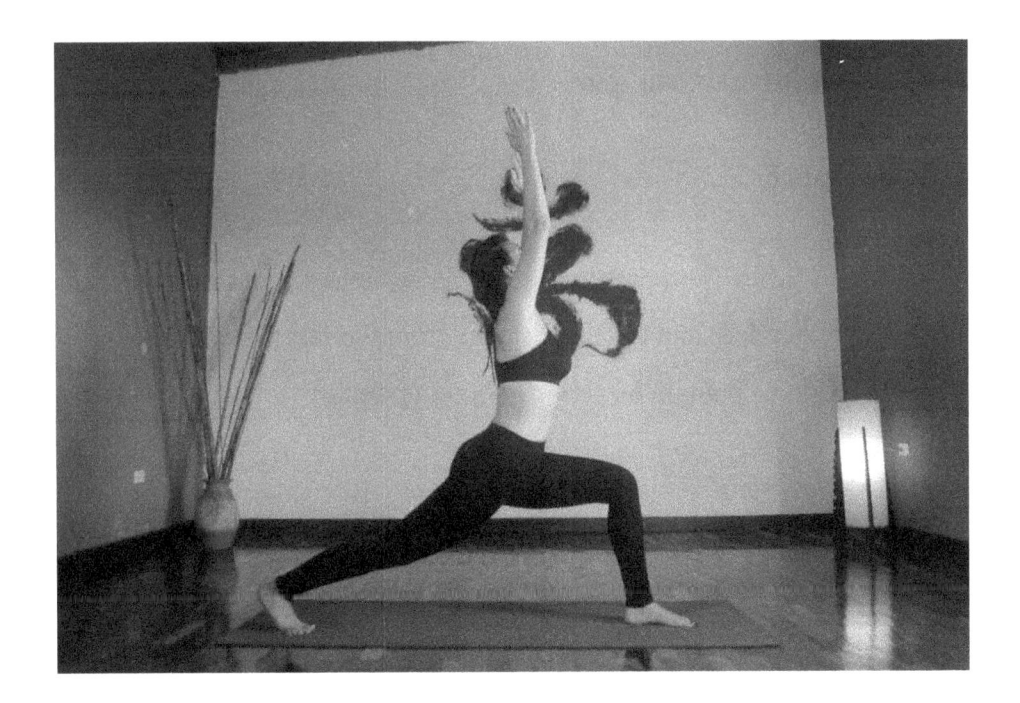

Chapter 5

Right foot goes forward, left foot is back a quarter of a distance, right knee flexes deeply, pay attention of not passing toes, hips rotated forward, both arms and elbows are extended high, it can be done joining both hands or to maintaining a separation between them, the important thing is to keep the arms fully extended and to focus the gaze on the top. Keep breathing slowly and deeply.

Benefits

- Strengthens thighs and legs
- Contributes to the burning of muscle fat
- Keeps the abdominal muscles active
- Test the resistance and will power
- Flexes the arms and spine

Recommendations

- If you suffer from problems in the knees make a variant (with both legs extended) and cut the distance from the feet
- If you have pain in the cervical focus a point of view on the horizon.

Boat Pose - Navasana

Chapter 5

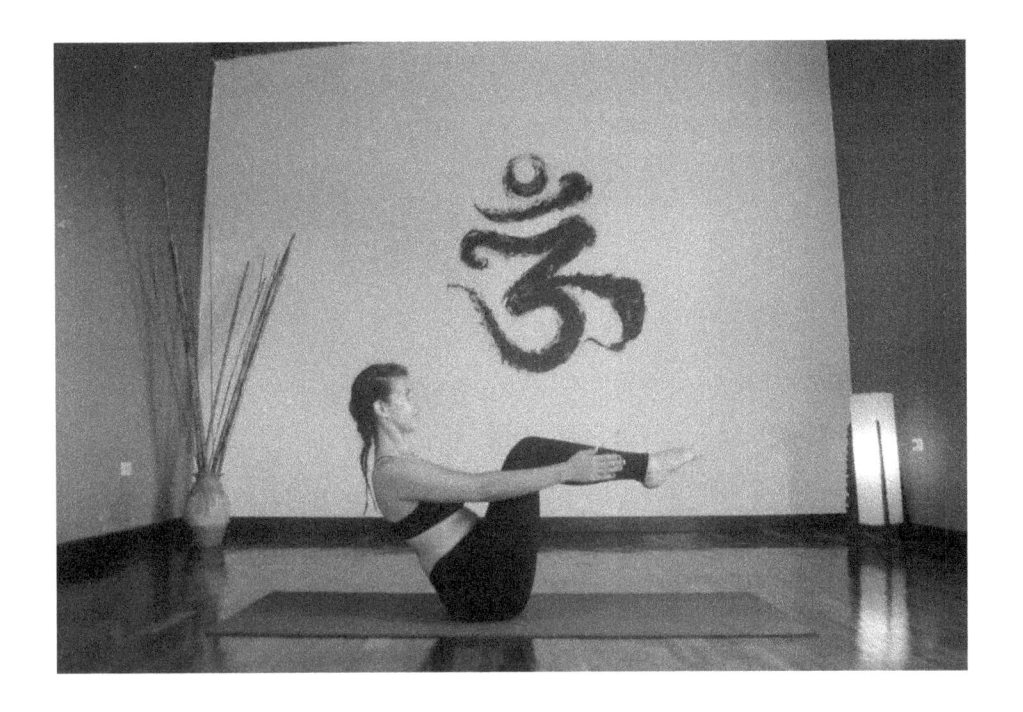

Sit on the mat with the knees bent to the chest, extend arms along, visualize the spine aligned and keep abdomen contracted. With the help of the conscious and slow breathing try to extend the legs little by little upwards, until be parallel with the ground. The position of the ship challenges the resistance of permanence in the postures.

Initial level, feet are separated from the floor with knees semi-flexed.

Intermediate or Advanced level, extend both knees and maintain.

Benefits

- Strengthens the abdominal walls and legs

Chapter 5

- Contributes to focus and determination
- Stimulates balance and balance
- Toning legs and abdomen.

Recommendations

- Do not give tension to the neck
- Contract the abdomen at all times
- If you feel weakness hug knees to chest with feet away from the ground and slowly try the variable that suits you.

Table Pose - Kumbhakasana

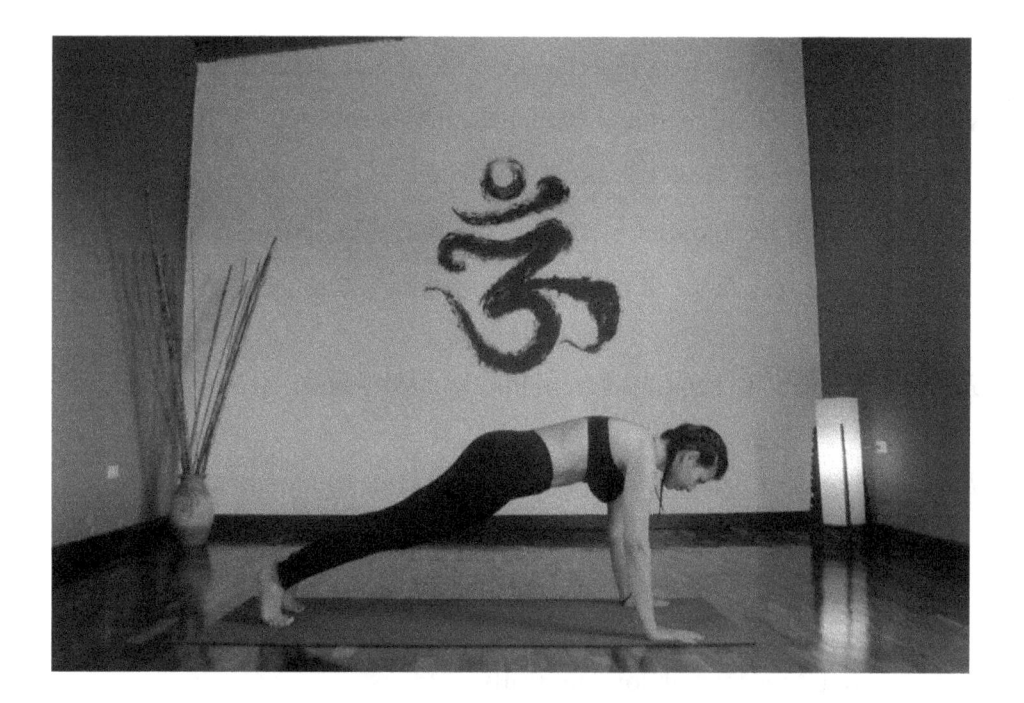

On the yoga mat support hands and feet distributing the weight between both hands and toes, the body is parallel to the ground, the focus is between both hands. It is important to keep the abdomen and buttocks contracted, strong arms and active feet. The breathing is rhythmic and continuous, always through the nose.

Benefits

- Strengthens the abdomen, buttocks and arms
- Stimulates the resistance of the body and mind
- Toning the chest and abdominal walls

Recommendations

- Do not drop the hip or raise the buttocks much
- Try as much as possible to keep the body in a straight line

Cobra Pose - Bhujangasana

Chapter 5

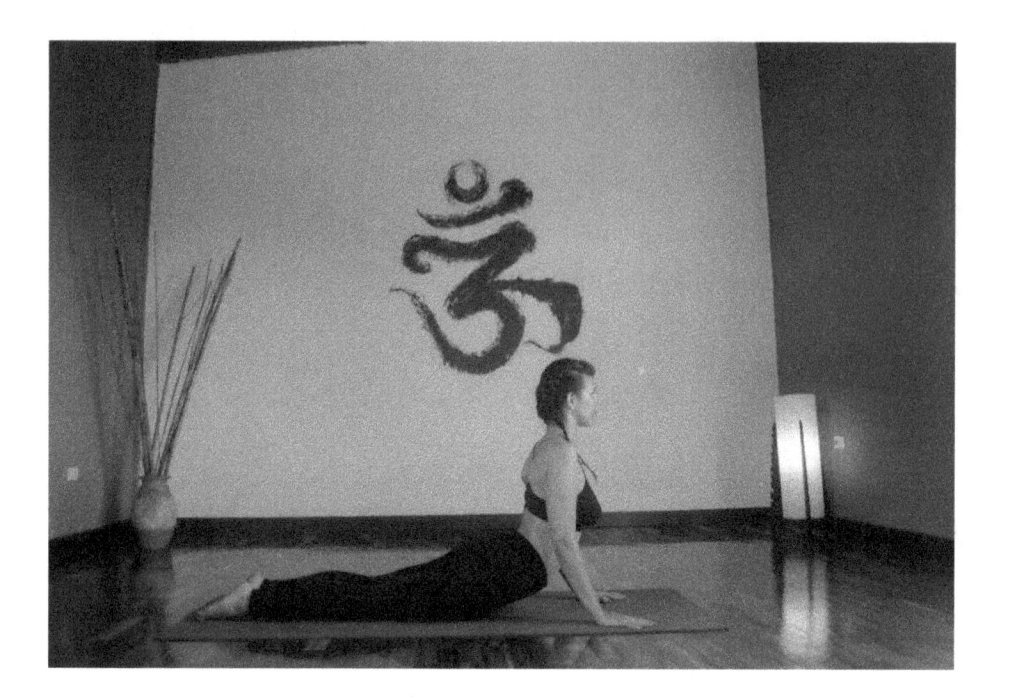

Lying face down on the yoga mat support firm hands on the floor near the ribs keeping the elbows closest to the body, slide forward, while the shoulders rotate back, the chest opens and the gaze is fixed on the horizon.

Benefits

- Tones up gluteus and legs
- Strengthens the vertebrae of the spine
- Stimulates the opening of the chest

Recommendations

- Keep the shoulders from ears
- Try to keep your feet as close together as possible
- Do not force the stretch of the spine

"Yoga is the practice of silencing the mind".

-Patanjali.

5.3 Yoga Poses for Balance

Variation in 4 Points of Support

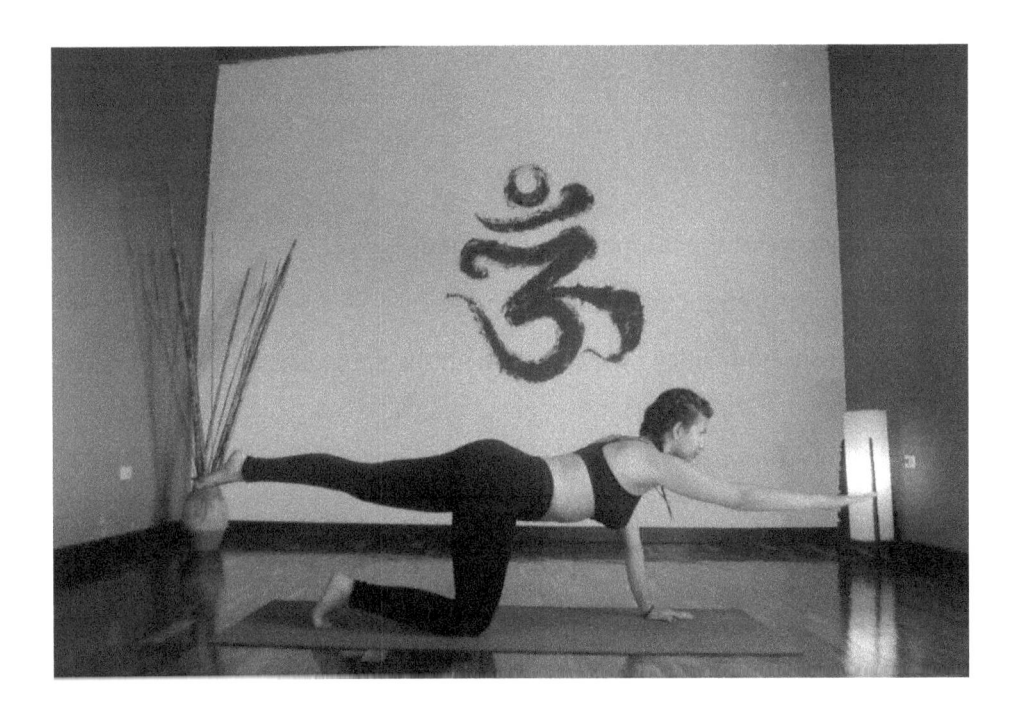

Lean on the yoga mat, hands and knees bent, align the hands just below the shoulders and knees under the hips with a slight separation, the toes remain active while the gaze focuses on a fixed point on the horizon. With a deep inhalation elevate the right leg and the left arm take care that these are parallel with the ground and fully extended. Stay in the balanced posture for 3 to 5 deep breaths.

Benefits

- Balances both sides of the body
- Contributes to concentration
- Strengthens muscles of the back and abdomen

Recommendations

- Take care of the alignment of the body
- Keep breathing controlled and paused
- Perform both sides of the body with the same dwell time

Cat and Cow - Bidalasana and Gomukhasana

Cow Inhale

Chapter 5

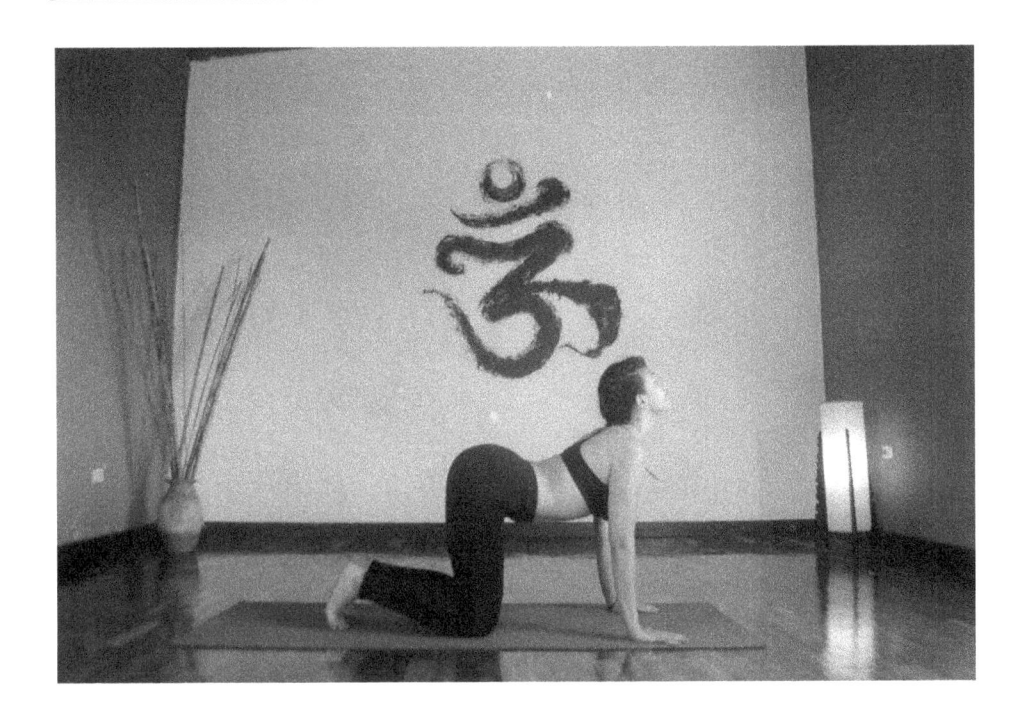

Cat Exhale

Chapter 5

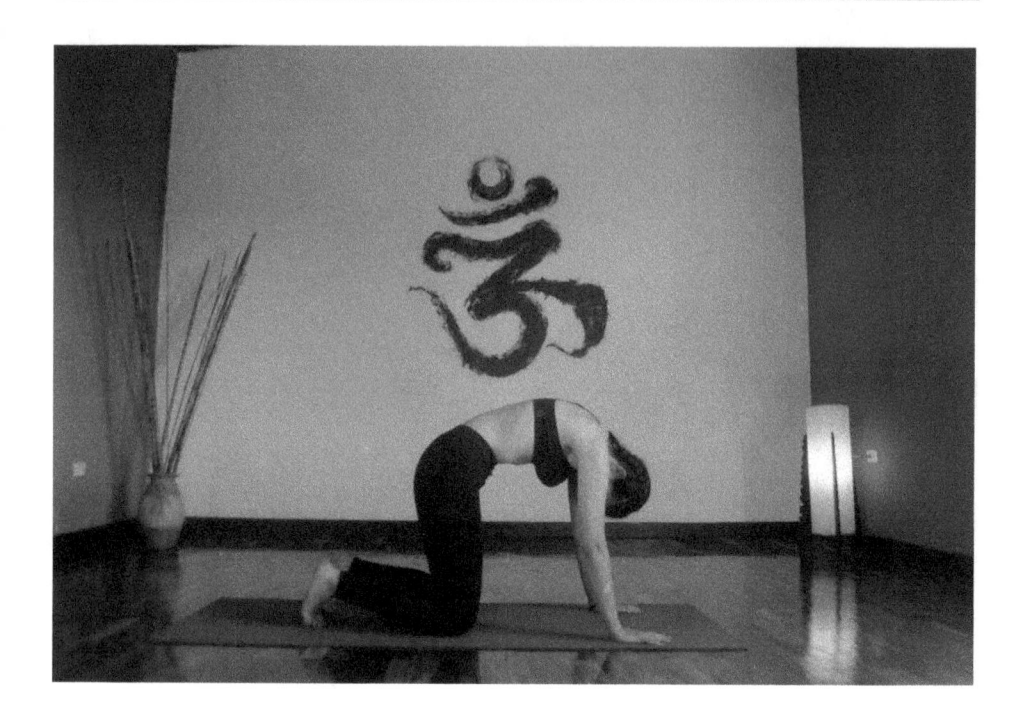

The hands rest firmly on the mat, opening the fingers like a fan, the hips are on their knees and the toes remain active.

With a deep inhalation, the shoulders are rotated backwards, the chest is opened, the gaze is raised high and the back arches, with the exhalation the head is tilted towards the floor, the spine is rounded and the gaze is directed to the navel. Repeat the sequence 5 times present in the breath.

Benefits

- Integrates breathing with movements

- Releases lumbar and cervical discomfort
- Strengthens the spine
- Toning thighs and arms.

Recommendations

- To care for the knees, use cushions under them
- Align shoulders on wrists and hips on knees
- Do the movements with pause and care.

Butterfly Pose - Baddha Konasana

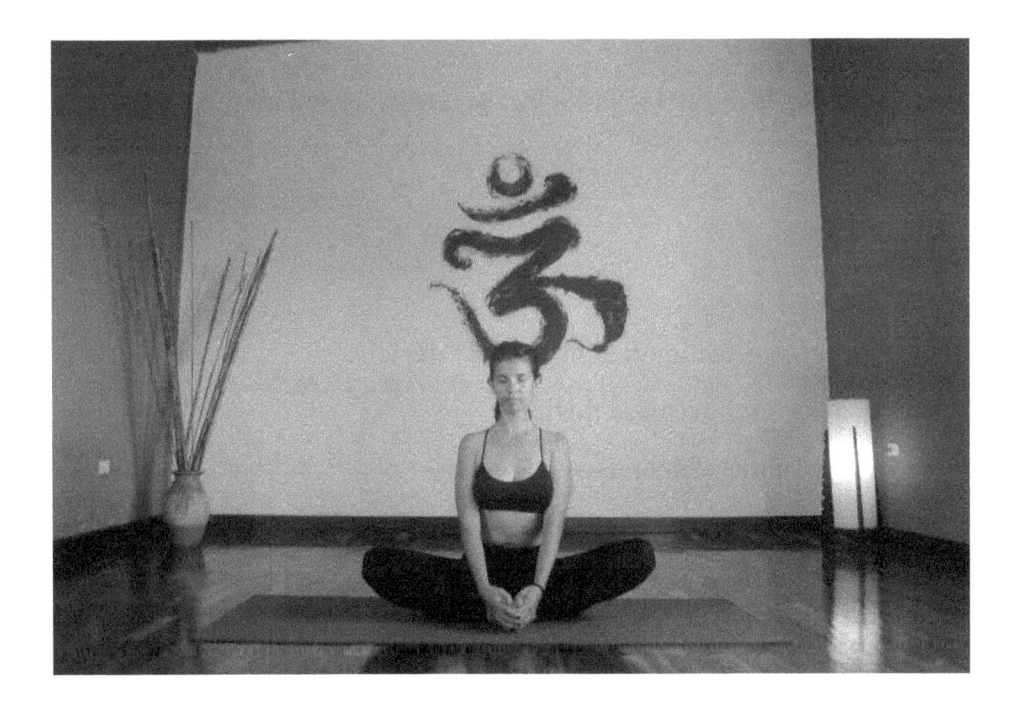

Chapter 5

Sit on the yoga mat with knees bent together with both soles of the feet. The spine is kept completely straight. The sole of the feet is taken with both hands and it is sought to rotate them upwards, the heels are kept as close as possible to the genital area, providing the opening of the hips. Take a deep inhale while the back seeks to bend forward, in this movement the forearms rest on the thighs, while the back seeks the ground.

Level 1: Stay in the posture with the spine straight.

Level 2: flex back forward.

Level 3: In forward bending with the chest touching the ground.

Note: Breathing is of vital importance, as it is what will allow us to deepen the movements.

Benefits

- Strengthens the internal muscles of the legs
- Makes your hips more flexible
- Aligns of the vertebrae with kindness
- Stimulates the sexual organs

Recommendations

- Pay attention to your tolerance levels

- Do not force the posture
- If you have lumbar pain, avoid forward flexion.

Sitting Half Spinal Twist Pose - Ardha Matsyendrasana

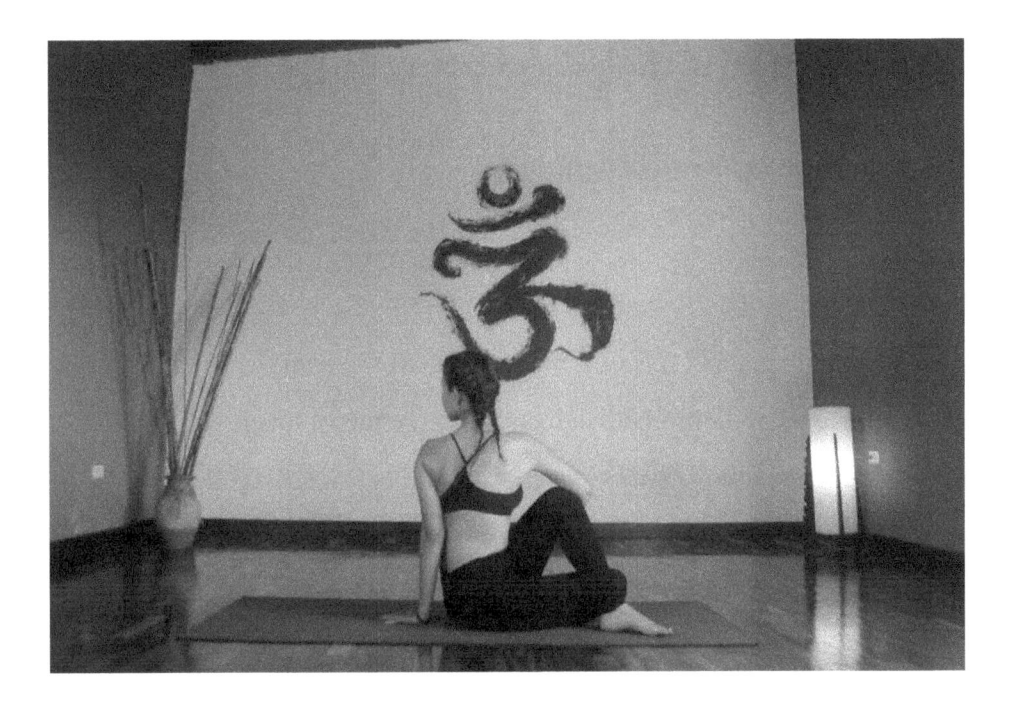

On the floor with the legs extended in front and the hands on the knees, the left knee is raised and flexed in coordination with the breathing. Following this, the right knee is flexed and brought under the left leg until the heel touches the outer face of the gluteus (both knees are flexed).

Then the left foot is passed outside the knee that is resting on the floor, slowly turning the trunk of the body to the left, doing a twist, right arm embraces left thigh.

Left arm goes behind the back, as close as possible to the spine. The head turns to the left and the look goes over the shoulder.

Repeat complementary side of the body.

Benefits

- Strengthens and relax all the muscles of the back
- Prevents and eliminate defects at the vertebral level
- Stimulates the nervous system
- Helps fight constipation.

Recommendations

- Perform the torsion with full attention and smoothness
- Maintain control of breathing
- Stay in the posture for 5 to 7 breaths.

Half Bridge Pose - *Setu bandha sarvangasana*

Chapter 5

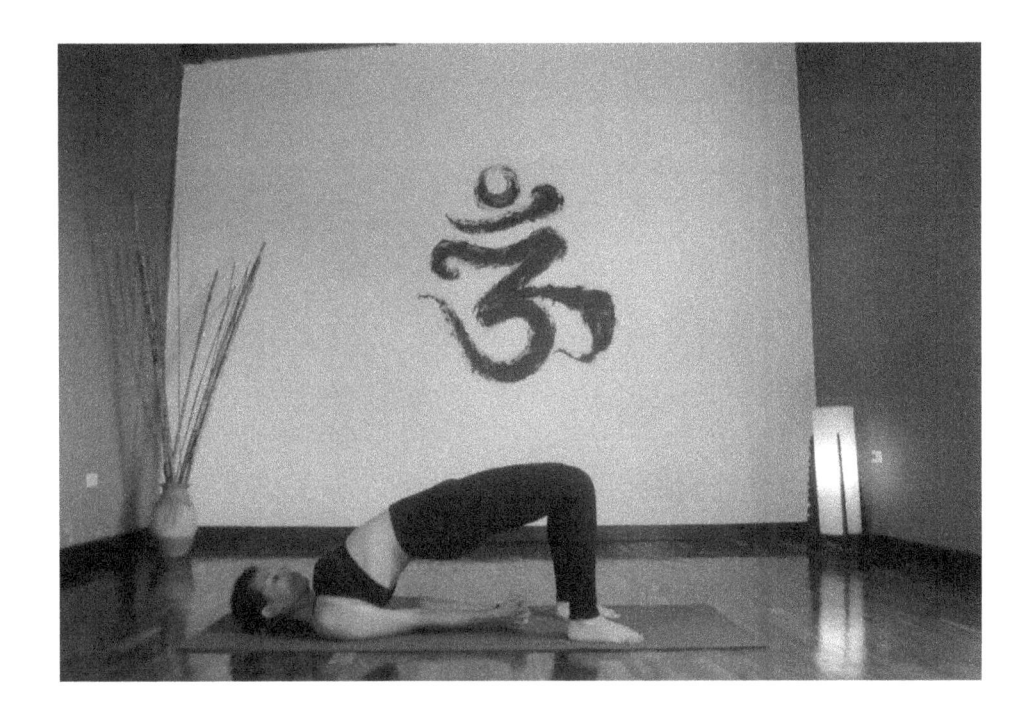

Supporting the back on the yoga mat, the knees are bent but this time the feet rest on the very close of the buttocks, the hands rest firmly on the mat, or if feeling comfortable in the posture, interlace hands behind the back without separate from the ground. Take a deep inhale while the buttocks and lower back are separated from the floor, the air is retained for a few seconds, when exhaling the body rests on the ground.

Benefits

- Strengthens lower back, buttocks and thighs
- Flexibility spine
- Tones abdominal walls and pelvic floor.

Chapter 5

Recommendations

- Pay attention to the conditions of your body
- Do not force neck or spine.

5.4 Yoga poses for Relaxation and Stimulation of Emotions

Head to Knee Forward Bend - Janu Sirsasana

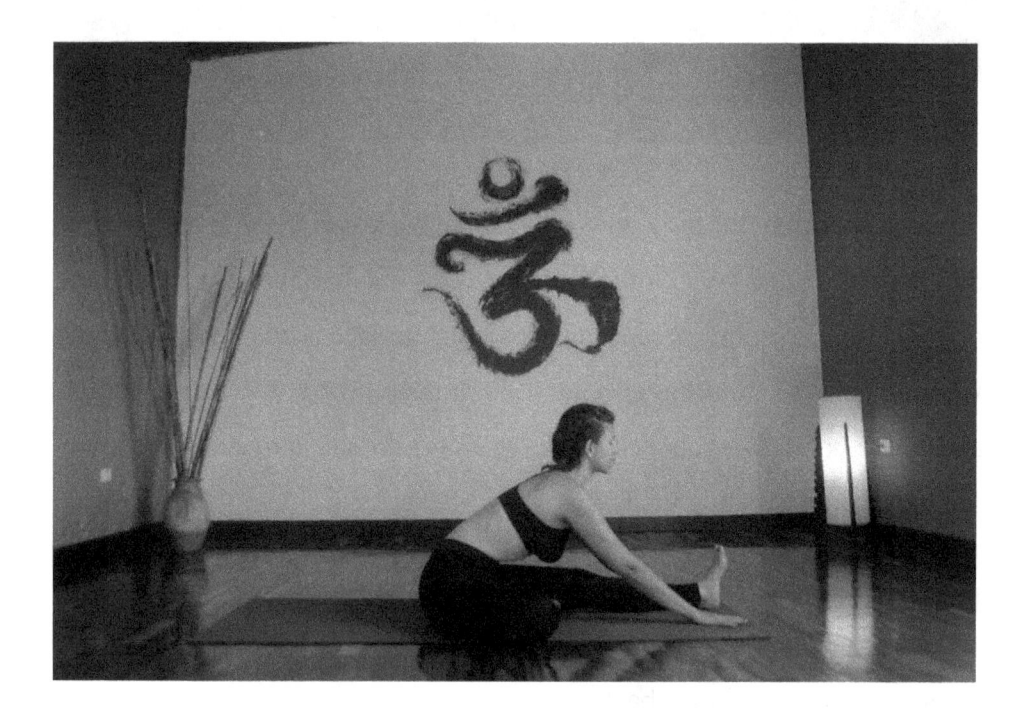

Sitting on the yoga mat with both legs extended and the back fully straight, bend the right knee and bring the sole of the foot close to the inner thigh take a deep inhale while the back of the body is leaning forward on the leg that remains extended With a slight pressure on the abdomen, the hands are extended to the sides of the leg and the eyes focus on the foot. The back should be kept as straight as possible and the breathing should be slow and deep.

Benefits

- Stimulates the sexual organs
- Contributes to the good digestion of food
- Corrects the posture of the spine

Recommendations

- Do not bend your back, try to maintain the straightness of the spine
- If you feel comfortable in the posture and you want to go deeper, extend the arms until the nose over the knee
- Maintain the posture of 5 to 8 deep breathing.

Wind Relieving Pose - Pavanamuktasana

Chapter 5

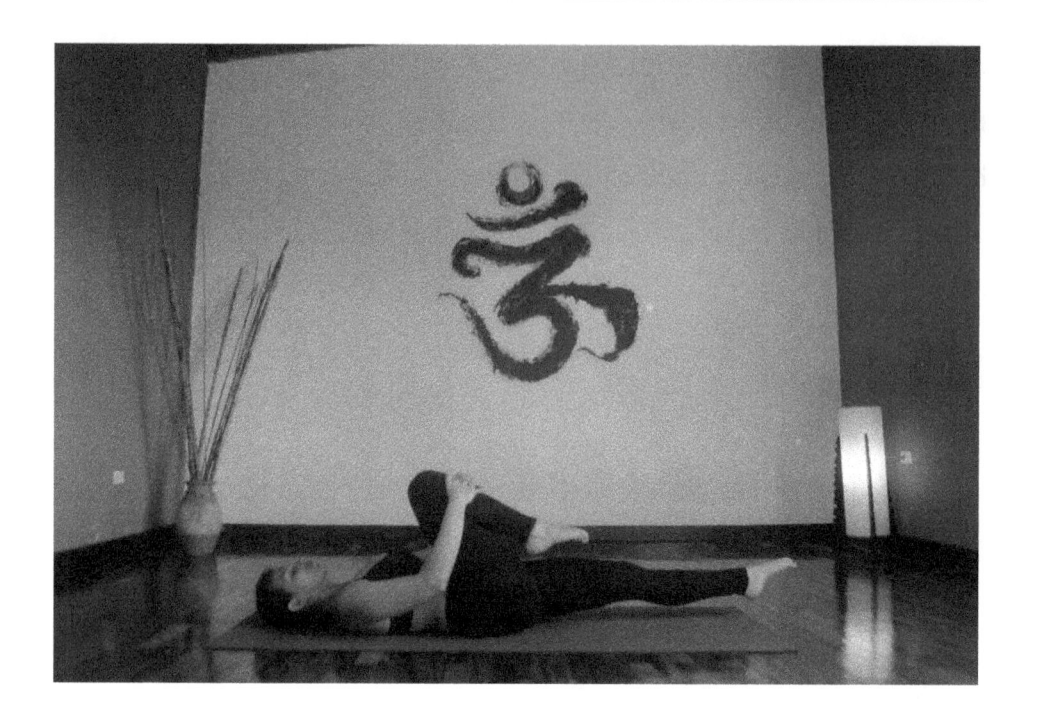

On the mat, lying on your back, flex both knees to the chest, hugging subtly, keeping your back, neck and head supported on the mat. The flexion of the right knee is maintained, while the left knee extends, the leg looks for the floor, but stays in the air a few centimeters from it, both feet stay in tip, the pressure in the abdomen is maintained with the strength of the arms. Release the position on the right side, perform the complementary side in the same way.

It is important that when you are working both sides of the body, you want to maintain the same number of breaths and the same variants.

Benefits

- Tone the abdominal walls
- Strengthen muscles and joints
- Stimulate the digestive system.

Recommendations

- If you feel tension in the neck, let the extended leg rest
- Keep your breathing controlled and paused.

Lying Down Body Twist - Vajrasana

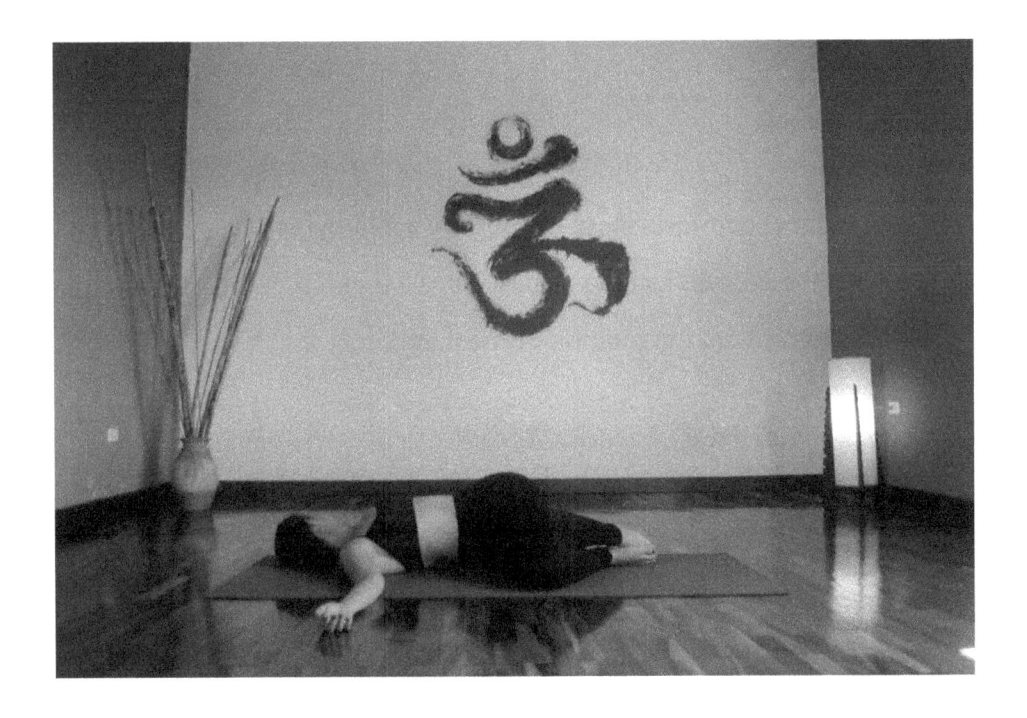

Following the previous position, keep the knees bent in the chest, this time drop both knees on the right side of the body while the arms are opened wide and the gaze goes on the left man performing a simple twist of the body. Maintain 7 to 12 breaths and perform the complementary side (drop knees from left side to look over right man).

Benefits

- Relieve discomfort in the lower back and neck
- Relax the nervous system
- Contribute to the stillness of the mind

Recommendations

- If you feel comfortable in the posture spread your legs in the twist
- Keep the posture as long as possible
- Be careful with the rotation of the neck

Legs Up The Wall Pose - Viparita Karani

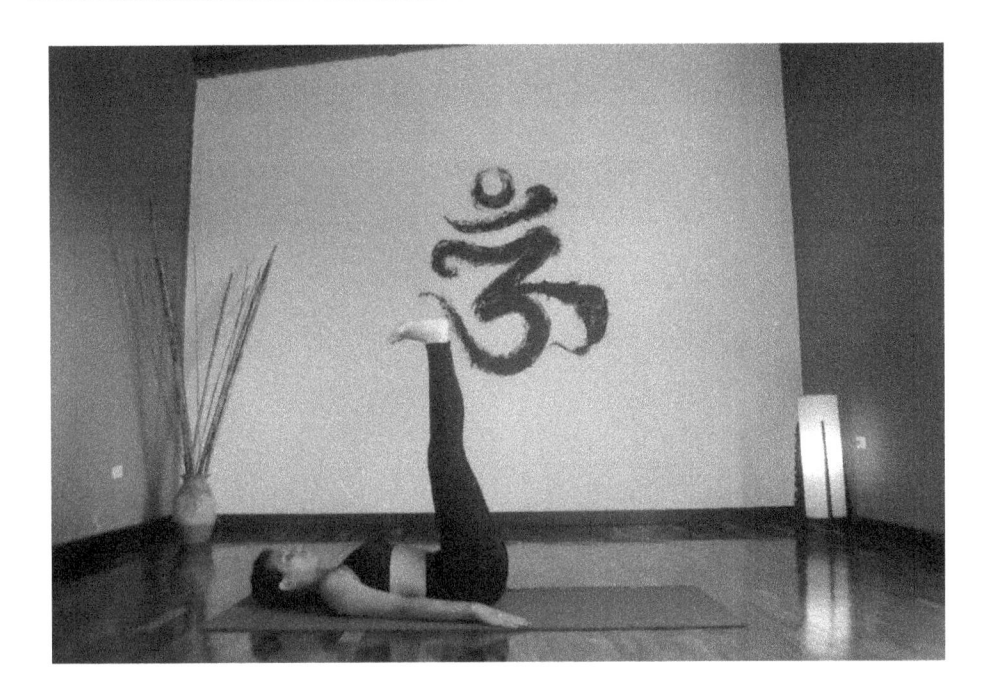

Lying on the back of the mat, bend the knees to the chest, support the hands next to the body and slowly extend the legs on top. They can help with a wall supporting the legs. Take care to keep your back, shoulders, neck and head resting on the mat, the gaze is fixed on the toes.

Benefits

- Stimulate the circulation of blood in the legs
- Strengthen the abdominal walls
- Encourages concentration
- Releases pain in the soles of the feet

Chapter 5

Recommendations

- If you feel discomfort when you fully extend your knees, semi flex them
- Do not separate shoulders from the floor
- Firmly support the hands next to the body.

Corpse Pose – Savasana

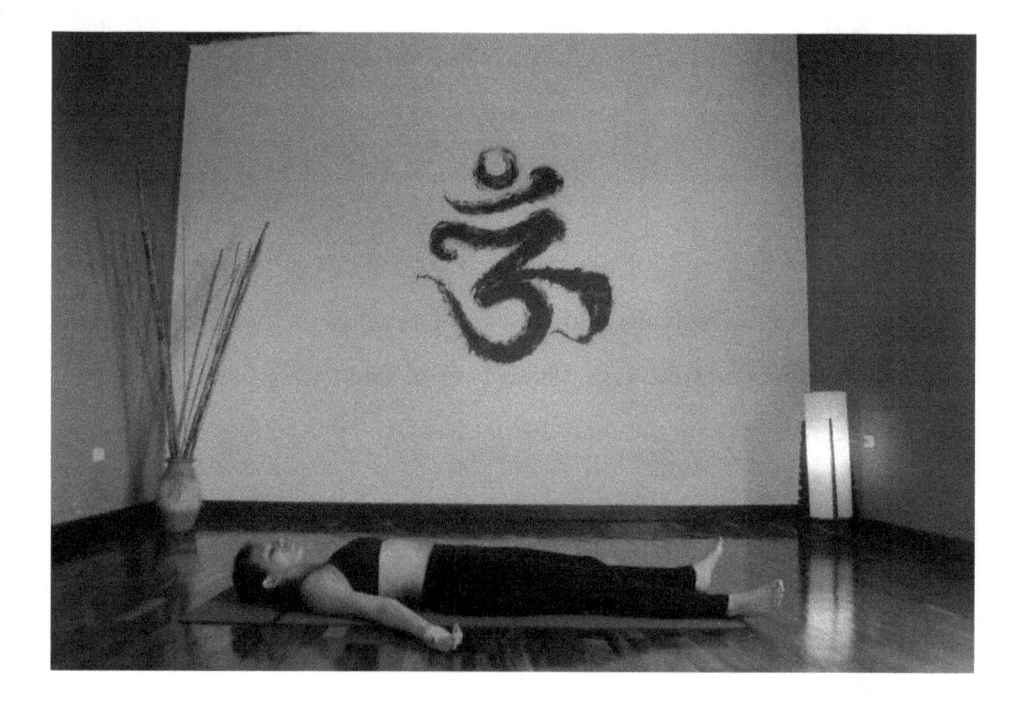

Lie comfortably on a mat, face up, allowing the body to relax completely. Feet naturally fall to the sides and are separated to the width of the hips, arms rest on the floor, hands are relaxed with palms facing up, there is no tension in the neck, nor the face.

It is inhaled by first filling the abdominal lower diaphragmatic part, filling the lower part of the lungs, in such a way that the diaphragm presses the abdomen and it tends to expand it. Then with the same inhalation, the intercostal middle part and finally the upper clavicles part are filled. They are held for a few seconds and the air is expelled slowly, the navel energetically seeks the spine. - repeat this breathing exercise throughout the practice, repeating the asanas 3 to 5 times.

Benefits

- Develop the alignment of each vertebra of the column
- Relax the body
- Encourages the concentration of the mind
- Increases lung volume and capacity.

Recommendations

- Use a rug, mat or yoga mat
- Please allow yourself relaxation in this pose
- Preferably keep eyes closed

Chapter 5

When these types of sequences are practiced in a continuous and fluid way, cleaning the body of impurities. These asanas have been ideally designed for curvy girls, as they tone the buttocks, hips and legs, strengthen the abdomen and help shape the figure.

Encourage and practice with enthusiasm, set goals and find the time to reach the objectives.

CHAPTER 6

Healthy Food for Yoguis

Chapter 6

6.1 Importance of a Balanced Diet

In the practice of Yoga, food is fundamental, since this is the fuel for an optimal life; The body needs the energy and nutrients that the food provides to perform all its functions and activities, such as: grow, develop, digest, breathe, think. Nutrients in foods are compounds that the body does not produce, so they must necessarily be obtained from the foods that are consumed. No food only contains all the nutrients in the right amount to meet the needs of the body. For this reason, it is important to eat varied and healthy foods.

In the philosophy of yoga food is vegetarian or vegan because of its diversity in colors, flavors, textures and healthy nutrients, respecting the right to life so that no meat or animal derivatives are ingested. It is for this reason that the Gunas are dynamically described, consisting of three streams: Sattva, Tama and Raja; Responsible for categorizing natural behaviors and phenomena; It is also used in Ayurvedic medicine as a system for diagnosing conditions and diets (According to Ayurveda, medicine and food are Sattvic, Rajasica or Tamasica, or the combination of the three) that represent the forms of balanced diet for all types of personalities.

6.2 The Gunas

The Gunas are understood as the qualities that sustain the universe, coming from the Teachings of Yoga, I mention this material with the

Chapter 6

objective of deepening the holistic benefits generated by the practice and a balanced diet. According to Hinduism, they are inseparable elements that combine in different proportions to form material objects. Guna is a Sanskrit word meaning "rope", "type" and generally "quality"; they are energies that act in our superficial mind and in our deep awareness, moving on a physical, emotional and mental level. These are also present in our behavior and feeding, according to the Bhagavah Ghita, a Guna is the most subtle quality of nature, and exists in all beings, translating as the balance in the coexistence we have with the entire universe.

Types of Gunas

1. Sattva: which symbolizes harmony, virtue, goodness, intelligence, imparts balance, peace, clarity, breadth and strength of love.

2. Rajas: on the other hand they are translated into energy, into excitement, and cause imbalance, greed, search for power and happiness outside of ourselves, dissatisfaction and characterize the nocturnal people.

3. Tamas: These are the heavier qualities, such as inertia, heaviness, drowsiness, ignorance, simplicity, disillusionment, laziness and block the spiritual awakening.

Now, how do we handle this information in our daily diet?

Chapter 6

Biologically we stimulate our consciousness and physical state, with the food we eat and the attitudes we have before life; among the benefits of the teachings of Yoga, is to generate serenity in our thoughts, elasticity, physical strengthening and awareness for health care.

If deserved attention is given to the foods that are consumed and in what way they are combined, it will be easier to classify them and create awareness of how we feed ourselves, since not only do we feed our body, we nourish our mind, as the Master Patanjali: "Let food be your medicine, let your medicine be your food"

Description of the foods of the 3 qualities (Gunas):

Sattvic foods are those that give us more vitality, good mood, tranquility, these help us maintain a better mental and physical balance, these foods must purify the body and clean energy channels, they must be natural and fresh foods, ideal To be consumed raw, boiled, steamed or lightly cooked.

For Example:

- ✓ Cereals (quinoa, oats, rice, corn, millet, among others) are ideal to provide our bodies with carbohydrates and amino acids that serve to synthesize proteins

- ✓ Legumes, grains and dried fruits (beans, lentils, chickpeas, beans, nuts, almonds, among others), high in protein and low in fat content
- ✓ Dairy products and butter, moderate consumption
- ✓ Aromatic spices or fine herbs (coriander, thyme, rosemary, oregano, basil, parsley, among others) are the ideal stimulus for our nervous and endocrine systems
- ✓ Fruits and vegetables, which provide our bodies with vitamins, minerals and fibers, also contain alkaline substances that work to keep the body clean and light
- ✓ Honey, molasses or maple syrup, are the sweeteners that are used in the sattvic diet.

Rajasic Foods: are bitter, sour, excessively spicy, salty, more baked and produce stimulation, excitement or addiction, among these are:

- ✓ Onions, garlic, radish, tea, coffee and all kinds of exciting things are included in this category, as well as highly flavored foods, chemical products, refined sugar (white), soft drinks, processed mustards, among others.

Tamasic Foods: is based on old, past, stale, overheated, consumed not important food, to fill and not to feed, and far from producing energy, consume our vital energy to be digested and leave us a feeling of tiredness, confusion and lethargy. . They produce toxins that generate imbalances.

Chapter 6

Among these, meat, fish, food loaded with fried foods, alcoholic beverages, marijuana and opium, drugs among others.

How do we integrate this information into our daily diet?

First we must identify that Guna is the one that influences our daily life, what kind of food we consume and how we eat it, what is our attitude (serenity, aggressiveness, heaviness), in this way we can adopt the necessary changes for a full and healthy life balancing the food that we bring to our table,

For example:

If you are an aggressive person and do not consume vegetables, but you love Yoga, you get the flexibility of your thoughts and it gives you the opportunity of a delicious fresh salad, I assure you that your stomach will thank you.

If you love meat or fish, it is not bad, maybe you just need to control the consumption of it, increase the vegetables, it will provide your body with a satiated state.

Remember, yoga is the union between our body, spirit and mind, the great teachers certify that the perfect diet is Satvica, a vegetarian diet, free from guilt, however, they are personal decisions, once we handle the correct information and the couple. Live with conscience and for the benefit of our mental and physical health. In Yoga, one believes faithfully in Ahimsa (nonviolence and respect for life); We are responsible for what we put into our mouths and also the way we say it, each step towards knowledge is an opportunity to transform habits and attitudes.

With these I do not mean to imply that it is a sin to have a few glasses of wine or to attend a barbecue with friends, rather, it is to give importance to the act of eating, to enjoy each bite and with grace and treachery to feed ourselves for the development of an entertaining life and healthy.

CHAPTER 7

Physical Transformation

Chapter 7

7.1 Yoga Integral Alternative for Weight Loss

Yoga, being an activity that involves every muscle of the body, is ideal to stimulate the loss of weight and the toning of the body with constant practice and continuous sequences. Yoga has overcome barriers of time, religions and ages, guaranteeing its practitioners the optimal functioning and integration of the mind, body and spirit. Developing people in a state of greater warmth and mental clarity, through knowledge, human values (Yamas and Niyamas), the practice of asanas (postures), the performance of pranayama (breathing exercises) and meditation (Pratyahara), strengthening the awareness and recognition of the subtle elements of the human senses.

Any time of the day or night, are suitable for the practice of yoga, just consider an intention and proceed to enjoy the multiple benefits that Yoga gives holistically. However, the great masters of this millennial practice like Patanjali, recommend starting the day with asanas, breathing exercises and meditation, taking advantage of the first rays of the sun to awaken the body and consciousness, in this way the body is given strength, coordination, balance and balance to start daily activities in a harmonious and efficient way.

One of the most popular sequences are the greetings to the sun which is the rhythmic continuity of several asanas, easy to memorize and even perform at home, in free time when you are at work, when waking up or

Chapter 7

dismissing the day, as well as they are also used to warm the body at the beginning of yoga classes and is recommended for anyone who wants strength, flexibility, physical, mental and spiritual well-being. The greeting to the sun is a sequence that consists of 12 simple asanas, synchronizing the inhalation and exhalation with each movement.

"It is through your body that you realize that you are a spark of divinity."

-B.K.S. Iyengar

Description of Greetings to the Sun A - Surya Namaskar A:

Elements to be used:

- ✓ Yoga mat
- ✓ Comfortable clothes
- ✓ Good Attitude.

Start standing on the upper edge of the mat, both feet spaced hip-width apart, legs extended, right spine, shoulders and facial muscles relaxed, arms at the sides of the body. Perform deep inspirations through the nose, release the air and relax the body, while creating a positive intention to practice.

1. Samasthiti Tadasa: standing, with the body fully erect, the palms meet in the center of the chest, the shoulders and face relax, inhaling and exhaling

Chapter 7

deeply the vertebral column is visualized in a straight line like a thread running through each vertebra.

2. Urdhva Hastasana: Take a deep breath while the arms extend over the head, open the chest and look up, lengthen the body as much as possible.

3. Uttanasana: Exhale, deep hip flexion forward, the crown of the head looks for the floor, the knees are extended, if you feel discomfort when extending the knees semi flex, while the abdomen rests on the frontal thighs, the hands can hold the calves, heels or the floor,

4. Ardha Uttanasana. Inhaling following the previous position, the gaze goes to the front, the hands rest on the calves or the floor with outstretched arms, the back lengthens.

5. Kumbakasana: inhaled both hands are supported on the floor, while the weight of the body is distributed in the palms of the hands and the tip of the feet the body is parallel to the floor, contracting abdomen and buttocks, the back stays in line straight.

6. Chaturanga: exhale, bending the elbows close to the ribs, the body leans slightly forward (semi flexion) or lies face down.

7. Urdha Mukha Svanasana. It is inhaled, the hands are between the hips, the insteps are held on the ground, the body is suspended in the air, while the chest expands and the head falls slightly backwards. If this variant is

very strong, try Bhujangasana (the cobra), lean on the floor, hands next to the ribs attached to the body, the shoulders rotate backwards, the expansion of the chest.

8. Adho Mukaha Svanasana. It is exhaled, the hands rest firmly on the floor, the elbows and knees extend, the coccyx rises high while making an inverted v with the body, the look looks for the navel.

9. Ardha Uttanasana. It is inhaled

10. Uttanasana. Exhale

11. Urdhva Hastasana. It is inhaled

12. Tadasana. Exhale

Benefits

- ✓ Stimulate body systems
- ✓ Promote flexibility and corporal dexterity
- ✓ Contribute to the concentration of the mind
- ✓ Offer strength, conditioning and resistance to the body

Recommendations

- ✓ Repeat the sequence as many times as possible

- ✓ Maintain a controlled breathing rhythm and synchronized with each movement
- ✓ Respect the conditions of your body.

7.2 Increased Self-Esteem: Trust and Security

The more you practice yoga, the greater the benefits. Really with the passage of time it is amazing what can be achieved with dedication and commitment; Yoga is a discipline that must be done daily to develop the maximum potentials that are held in the body, mind and spirit. Being able to control emotions and neutralize sensations is a fundamental part of life, as this guarantees happiness and well-being.

The positive thoughts, the confidence in the movements and the words are acquired little by little with each step that is advanced in practice as well as the security that develops with the actions. Mastering the body through breathing and achieving unimaginable postures is possible with the practice of yoga the body becomes flexible at the same time as the mind, creating unlimited possibilities and the sensations of being able to conquer fears, release the bonds of the mind and the attachments to the material.

CHAPTER 8

The Moment is Here and Now

Chapter 8

Living in the present is perhaps one of the greatest teachings of yoga philosophy, to appreciate the present moment when one awakens from consciousness through meditation, pranayamas and asanas. If not now when? It is one of the phrases that generate more vibrations. When? So that we postpone the wonderful things that can be done in the here and now with the best tools that are: the mind, the body and the spirit.

To thank even the most minute details of life, to contemplate time while walking with a pause honoring what we are, what we have and even what we do not have. Accept the turbulent thoughts and continue in search of solutions in what the yoga practice teaches us, relaxing the mind and the body.

Yoga is the motor that drives self-recognition by freeing us from labels, judgment and competition. Meditation techniques lead human consciousness in the rational study of past, present and future time, the practice of yoga stimulates faith in what is done and transforms it into beings of free souls developing the perception and authenticity of thoughts, words and Actions.

Experience the multiple benefits of yoga for you, fill your life with well-being and possibilities, there are no excuses. Your mind and your body will appreciate the initiative to start the practice of yoga.

Chapter 8

"When a yogi begins to meditate, he must leave behind all sensory thinking and all possessions, quieting the waves of feeling and the mental restlessness that arises from them, through the application of techniques that restore the power to control the unlimited supra consciousness of the mistress".

-Paramahansa Yogananda.

CHAPTER 9

Positive Aspects of Performing Physical Activities

Chapter 9

9.1 Positive Effects Provided by the Constant Practice of Yoga and Exercise

In the search to look healthy and beautiful, physical conditioning is the protagonist. The performance of yoga practices and psychophysical exercises contributes to the activation of the body by strengthening muscles and bones, stimulating self-esteem and even acts in a preventive manner against diseases and symptoms of aging. Physical activities teach you to live healthily and move forward with a balanced and resilient organism.

How to get a healthy body and a healthy mind?

Adapting to the daily routines a little training, optimism and discipline.

Health is the result of the will in action. Deciding to undertake a physical discipline that generates neuromuscular conditioning, stimulation of the senses, social interaction, body and mind training, are principles to ensure a healthy body and a healthy mind.

Tips:

- ✓ Identify what physical activity you like so you feel motivated to do it
- ✓ Start with the easiest and most comfortable thing you can do

Chapter 9

- ✓ Create routines for daily exercises such as: stretching, cardiovascular warm-ups, riding a bicycle, experiencing extreme sports, playing soccer, doing yoga, among others
- ✓ Add fruits, vegetables, cereals and nuts to your diet that allow you to gain energy
- ✓ Be persistent with the activities you decide to carry out

The realization of psychophysical activities such as exercise, are open doors for all people wishing to add balance and strength to their lives, that is why every day there are more people who join physical activities looking for wellbeing and the release of stress. Observe carefully what the universe reveals along the way and develop awareness for the acceptance and transformation of behaviors or habits with the aim of establishing a balanced, healthy and optimistic state.

The sympathy with others contributes considerably to the evolution of man and more and more people are in the world sharing their stories, experiences, hobbies, and the best content that is in them.

"Keeping the body healthy is our duty, otherwise we will not be able to preserve our mind strong and clear"

-Buddha.

Chapter 9

A healthy body guarantees the proliferation of positive thoughts and attitudes. The beginnings symbolize challenges for all but it is essential to identify an intention to undertake the paths of well-being.

The regular practice of exercises allows them to experience

- ✓ Cardiovascular resistance
- ✓ Physical and mental conditioning
- ✓ Better functioning of the internal organs and glands (heart, brain, stomach, among others)
- ✓ Muscular strength
- ✓ Resistance
- ✓ Flexibility
- ✓ Good mood
- ✓ Security and trust

Physical health naturally attracts emotional and mental health, developing receptivity in people, security and trust. What generates the increase of self-esteem and the best performance of the intellect, obtaining as a result that people can more easily comply with the demands of work, household chores and even relate to other people.

Keeping the body moving, the heart happy and the positive mind tones the physical, sensory, mental and communication skills. Performing activities of high physical and mental requirement allows the acquisition of good habits, enjoyment of health and long life.

9.2 Welfare and for the environment

The practice of yoga is a complementary activity of life, which has been shown to be beneficial in the prevention of diseases, rehabilitation of physical health and the development of thought by encouraging people to conquer the positive transformation of habits and behaviors.

The benefits generated by the practice of Yoga are convenient for its practitioners and their environment, since Yoga contributes to the mental health of each individual, generating receptivity and tolerance in the coexistence of people.

The practice of physical and mental activity allows people to enjoy well-being and good attitude, this thanks to the sum of positive thoughts and the release of stress.

The benefits of Yoga are almost immediate for people who commit themselves to this holistic practice.

Yoga allows the human being to inquire so much into his being through meditation that guides people to know each other better, respect their times, their needs, define their own interests, recognize strengths,

Chapter 9

accept weaknesses, detach from the results of actions and above all to serve others in a positive and compassionate way.

Many people are linked to yoga through songs (mantras), dances, social services (karma yoga) and studies of the sacred scriptures, each one is free to follow the steps of their preference. The important thing is to set goals of improvement and well-being, in order to contribute to the world and make the environment a better place for all.

There are many stories, experiences, hobbies or hobbies that can unite people, Yoga is an open door for anyone who seeks strength, balance and well-being. It is simply observing with attention what the universe reveals in the way and developing consciousness for the acceptance and transformation of behaviors or habits of life. The practice of yoga, enhances human values such as respect for life and Nonviolence -Ahimsa-. Developing in people compassionate love, free of competition among practitioners, the trial or the violent effort of the body to perform the postures -asanas-.

The sympathizing with the neighbor, contributes considerably to the evolution of man, and every time there are more practices of Yoga that are in the whole world sharing knowledge, cultures and the best content that is in them, without doubt, the sensibility of What this practice generates transcends boundaries and conquers compassionate love. Naturally the practice of yoga provides balance in the body, mind and spirit recreating the

Chapter 9

environment and our living conditions. Try it, just let yourself be surprised by yoga practice. It is really possible to heal the soul, transform habits and even evolve thoughts.

CHAPTER 10

Mindfulness

Chapter 10

The Awakening of Consciousness

The goal of yoga is to reach the infinite potential of the human mind and soul, and -as a practice-symbolizes the union of individual consciousness with divinity. This practice comprises different exercises that guide the strengthening of the body by performing a variety movements with intercalating postures or asanas, and conscious breathing techniques. Adding to this, yoga encourages disinterested service, mindfulness, compassionate love, the study of life and meditation.

Yogis and yoginis are spontaneous and nature-loving beings with immense sensitivity to details of everyday life, they develop the *mindfulness* of their acts and movements, showing themselves to the world as *free souls*, through the practice of *yoga*.

> *"Supremely successful man, Oh Arjuna!. Is he who disciplines his senses through the mind, with detachment and keeps the organs of activity fixed on the path of actions leading to union with divinity"*.
>
> Krishna.

Developing full attention in our lives is the fruit we reap by maintaining control over the mind, as it has the potential to contribute to the awakening of mindfulness: paying attention to thoughts, acts, emotions,

Chapter 10

bodily sensations, respiratory rate and our surrounding environment; Kabat-Zinn (1994) describes in *The Techniques of Stress Reduction Based on Full Attention* that: *"Paying attention in a particular way, as a purpose, in the present moment and without moral judgments"*. This introduction to mindfulness promotes effective management of mind and body through meditation and yoga practice to develop mindfulness in our own lives.

The mind is the sum of all accumulated conditioning, it is time, past and future, expressed through desire, emotions and behavior, is also recognized as painful memories that manifest in attachment, resentment, violence and joy. Yoga allows to recognize the potential within each of us, to fall in love with yourself and to dominate the realm of the mind for personal growth.

Each of us has the potential to achieve a *victorious life*. Integrating daily routines with the *practice of exercises*, meditation techniques that guide the *mindfulness* and activities that encourage contact with nature; discipline and effort will bring us closer to holistic well-being and gratitude to life.

Exercise:

Begin by breathing slowly, in a comfortable position, allow yourself to feel your body sensations, identify daily responsibilities, the tasks pending, the discomforts and restlessness of the mind and so on. As you

Chapter 10

read these lines, feel the present, release the tension of the shoulders and watch as thoughts come and go, maintain the awareness of each inhalation and each exhalation, experience the present, prioritizing your thoughts, create solutions to adversity, trust in your sound judgment and potential. Relax every muscle in your body inhaling and exhaling and in time, you will understand what is inside. Observe. Listen. Pay attention.

You realize that if you can, when you try. Your curvy body is ready to experience the positive benefits generated by yoga practice and your mind is ready to enjoy the full attention of the here and now.

We are dormant opportunities,

Come out and live,

Here and now.

General recommendations

Encourage yourself to enjoy yoga as a tool of well-being, stimulation and release of stress. Flowing with your body accept your curves, contours and measures, sensitizing the senses and awakening the channels of connection with the universe.

- ✓ Find the time

Chapter 10

- ✓ Find in you the greatest motivation to make your goals and dreams possible
- ✓ Commit to highlighting the best of yourself
- ✓ Practice yoga at any time, but do it.

"The true yoga is not about the shape of your body, but about the shape of your life. Yoga is not realized, it is lived. Yoga does not care what you have been; he cares about the person you are becoming".

-Aadil Palkhivala.